WITHDRAWN
Environmental
Health

A Paradox of Progress

John Phillips, Jr.

*State University of New York,
Sullivan County Com*

D1362309

wcb
WM. C. BROWN COMPANY PUBLISHERS
Dubuque, Iowa

CONTEMPORARY TOPICS IN HEALTH SCIENCE SERIES

Consulting Editor
ROBERT KAPLAN
Ohio State University

Exercise, Rest and Relaxation—*Richard T. Mackey, Miami University*

Alcohol: Use, Nonuse and Abuse—*Charles R. Carroll, Ball State University*

Reducing the Risk of Non-Communicable Diseases—*Wesley P. Cushman, The Ohio State University*

Drug Abuse: Perspectives on Drugs—*Robert Kaplan, The Ohio State University*

Smoking—*John T. Fodor, and Lennin H. Glass, San Fernando Valley State College*

Mental Health—*James C. Pearson*

Consumer Health—*Miriam L. Tuck, The City University of New York*

Venereal Disease: A Social Catastrophe—*Stephen J. Bender, San Diego State College*

The Human Body: Anatomy and Physiology—*Charles R. Schroeder, Memphis State University*

Environmental Health: A Paradox of Progress—*John Phillips, Jr., Sullivan County Community College*

Sex Education—*Robert Kaplan, The Ohio State University*

This book is dedicated to nurturing the quality of "humanness" in man. It is with the belief that the value of humanness is the prime value—and that the decisions regarding population and pollution must be made relative to human worth and human values—that this book was written.

Foreword

Health education is more than the primary phase of preventive medicine. Beyond the prevention of disease and the amelioration of health problems is its positive design to raise levels of well-being and liberate man's potential. Directly and indirectly it enables the individual to function most productively, creatively, and humanely.

One needs health to become educated and one needs education to develop and maintain health. Nor can one make full use of his education without it. Health is vital to the attainment of goals but we cannot preoccupy ourselves seeking it or in our obsession we shall fail to integrate all aspects of our development and performance. Health is a means to ends—the ends valued by the individual and society. Favorable modifications of health behaviors are essential to the attainment of these ends.

Contemporary Topics in Health Science offers a new and individualized format. Students and instructors can select and utilize those topics most revelant or most pertinent for the time available. Independent and class study, separately or concurrently, are enhanced by their organization. In this form they also provide greater opportunity to correlate health with other subjects.

Each book offers an up-to-date realistic discussion of currently significant health topics. Each explores its area in somewhat greater depth, with less trivia, than found in many textbook chapters. But they are designed to do more than merely present information. Within each are to be found more than partial explanations of facts. They are written by authors ranked by their professional peers as an authority in his field. They encourage the exploration of ideas, development of concepts, identifying value judgments, and selecting from a range of alternatives to enhance critical decision-making.

ROBERT KAPLAN, PH.D.
Consulting Editor

Preface

This book is about man and his environment. It is thus a book about you and me and the impact of our living processes on the quality of the environment. It is meant to be a very personal book.

Intended primarily for college students in health courses designed for both majors and non-majors, it may in addition be used as a supplementary text in such basic freshman courses as Science Survey and General Biology. Presenting an overview of the entire environmental crisis, the book can also be used advantageously for introductory reading in the many newly-emerging courses centering on man and his environment.

The book's content and design have evolved from the author's approach to the topic of environmental health in the actual classroom situation. This approach has been developed with two major factors borne in mind: the needs of the students as sensed during classroom discussions; and the realization that the ultimate solution to the environmental crisis lies in how each individual responds to the problems of overpopulation and pollution.

It is hoped that this work will mark a fruitful beginning of the student's realization that he has responsibilities as an "individual man" in solving the environmental crisis. The student should note, however, that the book raises more questions than it answers. On many of the issues there are no clear-cut answers. An attempt has been made, nonetheless, to delineate these issues and to stimulate the student's thinking so that he will be challenged to engage in further inquiry. If the student is to gain a full understanding of the complexity of the problems relative to economics, cultural values, governmental functions, natural processes and the very quality of man's daily existence on the planet, further inquiry is essential.

This author is indebted to Robert Kaplan, Ph.D., for his suggestions and guidance, and also to my wife Sarah for her encouragement and assistance.

JOHN PHILLIPS, JR.

Contents

Introduction

For perhaps one-half of its existence the planet Earth lay lifeless and barren. At an unknown point in history simple life forms appeared and man's evolution began. This book is about man and the impact of his presence and activities on the quality of the planet's environment.

Many have questioned the soundness and worth of man's intrusions into the natural processes of the environment. One such person has been Mr. Edward Pogarsky, a former student, who expressed his concern in the form of the following poem:

i am the sea

In the beginning,
God created earth.
The earth was dry and barren.

God saw this,
and He was moved to tears
In his tears He conceived me.

i am the sea
i am alone

God said to me, "If you will
worship me I will give you the
sun which will warm you.
And I shall give you the wind
to sooth you at night."

i said "yes"
for i was alone
and i was afraid.

1

Then God stretched out
His hand and gave me the light
i craved so badly. He gave
me the wind,

and i was Happy
for i was not alone

However, as time went by
i grew complacent. i thought
myself more powerful than God.
i commanded its wind and sun
alike to worship me instead of
God.

"Worship me not God," i said
to the Sun, or i will flood
your body

"Worship me," i commanded
the wind, or i shall overpower
you and engulf your breezes.
They obeyed, for they were afraid.
i was elated with the power that
was invested in me

God seemed far away

I was master,
I was God of all that I surveyed

God saw this, and He was angered
In a vision He appeared, and spoke
these words.

"You have set yourself up as a
higher divinity than Me. This is
a sin. For this sin I shall cast
three plagues on you. You will be a
whim of the elements, and a scorn of
time."

Out of my bowels came the plants,
then came the animals, then came
the deadliest plague of all . . .

Man

i saw man burn the plants and kill
the animals.
i cried out to God in pain to halt
man's inhumanity
But he paid no heed to me

i have seen civilizations
rise and fall.
And when there are no more
civilizations, and no more men
i shall still suffer

For i am the sea

i am alone

EDWARD POGARSKY

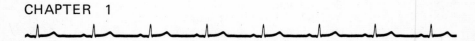

CHAPTER 1

Man's Environmental Dilemma

> *If we only knew what it were about, perhaps we could get about it better.*
> —A. LINCOLN

Man, since his emergence onto the grassy savannahs of Africa more than a million years ago, has always been engaged in three basic conflicts: with nature, his fellow man, and himself. The environmental crisis presently facing man brings him into simultaneous conflict with all three—a battle that may very well test man's ability to survive his own actions.

It's Your Dilemma

The environmental crisis cannot be classified as a dilemma that has its solution solely in scientific theory or modern technology. Its solution certainly does not lie solely in political expediency or economic readjustments. Nor does the solution rest within the realm of any specific discipline or manner of expertise. The solution rests squarely with *you*—the whole man, the organism with the capacity to function in a unique manner, not predetermined by genetic inheritance or history, not determined by scientific advances or available technology, but rather as determined by you, the integrated organism functioning within the framework of a philosophy of life involving values, judgments, decisions and actions, in relation not only to the natural elements but to all other living things also.

Man must consider all these factors in reaching a solution to his environmental crisis. His disregard for "wholeness" or ecological perspective has been the cause of man being faced with this crisis.

The Paradox of Progress

The problem of environmental crisis is not a new one. Thomas Malthus in 1798 wrote of a concern for the possible ill effects of expanding population on the welfare of mankind. History indicates clearly the smoke pollution problem encountered by the Romans during the development of the empire. Since the beginning of time, man's survival and well-being have been challenged by disease organisms borne by air, water, soil, as well as by vectors and other forms of environmental enemies.

Man, in attempting to meet and raise himself above and beyond this challenge, exhibited a strong drive to build and create and at the same time to dominate, destroy and exploit. Within the delicate balance of these forces, man has created his present environmental dilemma.

This dilemma in "delicate balance" may be referred to as the "paradox of progress." In prehistoric time man first made progress by using nature's fire, stones, plants and animals to meet his needs and by the time of Aristotle had developed a sort of "unlimited confidence" in the human mind. But environmental life was relatively simple, could be easily perceived and thereby managed.

With the growth of classical science man learned to put the new information to use, thus paving the way for the Industrial Revolution. At that point environmental life became more complex but nevertheless remained within the framework of the human mind's realm of reason and could still be managed. Thus the two opposing forces remained somewhat in balance.

However, beginning at the turn of the twentieth century, the rapid advances in modern science overpowered the mind of man. The five senses could no longer cope with the new forces introduced into the environment. Man had to adapt to new ideas relative to life, speed, distance, temperature and force before he could fully understand their potentials or limitations. Environmental life thus moved out of the "practicality" framework of the human mind and a degree of manageability consequently was lost. The loss of this manageability eventually brought man to this present state of ecological crisis.

A Technology Gone Wild

Examples of what appears to be this loss of manageability—technology on a rampage—are many and become more evident every day. The massive November, 1965 "blackout" which covered 80,000 square miles of the northeastern United States is one of the more startling manifestations of this situation. Consider the potential danger to the affected human population if the electric power failure had continued for a prolonged period.

Man and his environment are also experiencing such problems as radiation escaping from nuclear testing, the peaceful use of atomic energy, pollution of land, air and water, and rapidly expanding population.

Each of these problems will be dealt with separately, in the chapters that follow, in an attempt to highlight each of the critical issues. In so doing there is the danger of the loss of ecological perspective so necessary to a full understanding of the overall problem. The reader must constantly keep in mind that man lives and functions in an ecosystem (in a state of mutual relations with other organisms and their environment) and that as the centuries have passed, the ecosystem has become more complex, more sophisticated, more "man manipulated," until today it is difficult to differentiate between the constructive and the destructive forces within the system. The perspective one must take as he focuses on each of these problems offers evidence as to the many faces of the problem and to the complexity of the dilemma.

CHAPTER 2

The Ecosystem
and Man

Do we propose to live on the this planet in symbiotic harmony with our environment? Or preferring to be wantonly stupid, shall we choose to live like murderous and suicidal parasites that kill their host and so destroy themselves.

—ALDOUS HUXLEY

Man and all other organisms on the planet Earth live in a closed system, a biome. Photographs taken from the moon give clear evidence of the earth's desolate isolation and limited facility.

The ecosystem of man is limited to the planet Earth and its atmosphere, which extends approximately seven and one-half miles upward. Within the confines of the ecosystem lie all the elements known to man: the storms, the air, the water, the soil and all other living things.

The Natural Forces of Work

Some knowledge of the two fundamental laws of thermodynamics is essential to an understanding of the implications of man's functioning in a closed system. The first law concerns the "conservation of energy" and supports the fact that energy can be neither created nor destroyed. However, energy is constantly undergoing the process of distribution. The second law deals with this distribution factor, to the effect that energy direction is from an order structure to a disorder structure. Order is related to usable energy (more concentrated in form) and in the process of being used (work) it becomes less ordered (less concentrated in form).

Consider the following example: Man consumes sugar. This is energy in a concentrated form (an order structure). The sugar arrives at the cells and energy is extracted from its chemical bonds to meet the requirements for various life processes and functions. The energy thus becomes less ordered, even to the extent that some is rendered less

7

usable (as in heat radiated by the body). As a result the fraction of energy available for use is constantly being lessened.

There are methods, both biological and technological, for reconcentrating dispersed energy, a form of recycling. Though no method is completely efficient, this does not pose the major problem. The major problem factor in our environmental crisis is based upon man's nearly complete disregard for environmental cycles coupled with his wasteful use of natural resources.

The Cyclic Processes

From the moment man is conceived, he places demands on the environment. He requires air, water and food, and must eliminate wastes.

Man as a creature is not foreign to the earth. The process of evolution described by Darwin "fitted" him to the environment—he became part of it, a functional part, yet a mere phase in an overall plan of life.

Man is a conglomerate of the elements: carbon, oxygen, hydrogen, nitrogen and others. He does not have sole exclusive possession of these elements. Their origins lie somewhere in the distant past. Man merely has them for a short period of time in the many compounds that form various cells of the body. These same elements passed time and time again through various life cycles—perhaps once in a blade of grass, in an earthworm or a bird, or even in another human form.

In considering cyclic processes it is evident that what are one organism's wastes may serve as subsistence for yet another organism. Plants are fully capable of using organic wastes from animal life to produce plant protein. The carbon dioxide given off by animals supplies plants with raw materials necessary to the process of photosynthesis which in turn supplies animal life with available energy in the form of food and even restores vital oxygen to the atmosphere.

Consider man, who requires food, air and water and who must dispose of liquid, solid and gaseous wastes, in the following simple closed system—a biome where man and algae cycle various compounds in support of one another:

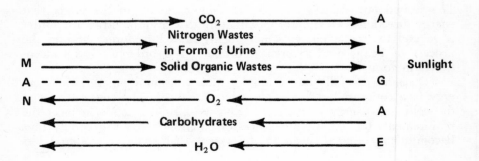

This system remains functional provided no shortages or over-balances occur. For example, an overconcentration of phosphates in the human wastes as part of the preceding cycle could cause the algae vegetation to smother in its own fecundity and so bring the cycle to an abrupt end. Any overbalance holds a disaster potential for such a cycle. A view of this cyclic process in the context of the larger ecological system will find the same basic problems existing.

The overabundance of man on planet Earth, his activities and the wastes resulting from those activities have served to tip the ecological scales. The dead lakes and ponds, the polluted air and water—even the quality of life for creatures struggling against extinction of their species furnish ample evidence. Man, too, is engaged in a struggle for survival that challenges the very quality of his daily life and perhaps even life itself.

The Effluence of Affluence

Modern man lives in a disposable world of "'no return bottles," throw-away items and elaborate packaging. He functions as if the world's natural resources were unlimited. He is infinitely more of a threat to the environment than was more primitive man. He requires, uses, and produces more waste.

Consider just one aspect of modern man's production, distribution and consumption patterns. In any supermarket, for example, the enormous number and variety of disposable items give clear evidence of man's *unnecessary* intrusions on the balance of nature. Specific example of this intrusion is the untold variety of disposable paper products such as paper cups, paper containers (as used for milk), food packaging—and so on and on!

The production of paper products requires the use of raw materials derived from steadily diminishing forest reserves. Cutting down these trees has great significance, since, in addition to the depletion factor, it clearly interferes with the cyclic process of carbon dioxide absorption and oxygen production. One acre of beech forest yields 1,500 pounds of pure oxygen a year, while removing 2,000 pounds of carbon dioxide. The trees also serve to hold the soil in place, and provide food and shelter for birds, squirrels and many other forms of wild life.

Each Man's Decision

Throughout the processes of production, distribution and consumption of any product, not just paper products, raw materials are used and pollutants produced. The question is, can man continue to produce "disposable" or nonessential items in the face of the growing environmental crisis? Can man continue to afford the production of an "oversized, gadget-loaded" automobile that produces more power than needed and pours out copious amounts of pollution while in in the process of devouring quantities of raw materials? Can man learn to function with a more practical vehicle that can be built and operated with a minimum of raw materials and so be not only less of a drain on raw materials but also less productive of pollutants?

With the expanding population and rising pollution levels taking place in a closed ecological system, obviously something has to give way. How man will ultimately handle this problem is questionable, but it remains obvious that any solution must rest with *each man's* decision as to how he will function within the ecosystem of his world.

That it is a complex situation was pointed out by Frederick Wilhelm Neitzsche (1844-1900) when he wrote: "Man shapes his own future, and that as well by what he does as by what he fails to do."

In what man will do or fail to do in relation to his environment lies the answer to the many questions regarding his future destiny.

1. Some of the proposed solutions to the problem of energy conservation and energy exchange in the environments hinge on the use of cyclic processes whenever possible. Consideration has been given to cycling collected garbage into highly efficient incinerators to serve as fuel for the heating of municipal buildings, etc. Waste paper which contains cellulose has been fed to cattle in the place of hay. Consider the potential for reusing materials in our society and develop some probable plans for such action.
2. Develop a documented (footnoted) essay reacting to the question and statement by Aldous Huxley at the beginning of this chapter.
3. Can you describe the relationships in more than one ecosystem? Write out as many as you can.

The Population Crisis

> *The power of population is indefinitely greater than the power in the earth to produce subsistence for man.*
> —THOMAS ROBERT MALTHUS

The decade of the '70s has arrived. William and Paul Paddock have forecast *FAMINE—1975!*[1] The world population continues to grow at the rate of 2 births per second; over 170,000 new individuals begin life on planet Earth each day.

In contrast, the earth's land mass remains the same, some 52 million square miles, of which only about one-third is habitable. Population density continues to increase. In 1930 the population density was 40 persons per square mile; today there are 63 persons per square mile and by the year 2000 the projections are for 142 persons per square mile.

Malthus Recognized the Problem

Thomas Robert Malthus, as early as 1798 took focus on the problem when he wrote in his paper "An Essay on the Principles of Population," the following:

I think I may fairly make two postulata.
First, that food is necessary to the existence of man.
Secondly, that the passion between the sexes is necessary, and will remain nearly in its present state.
These two laws ever since we have had any knowledge of mankind, appear to have been fixed laws of our nature; and we have not hitherto seen any alteration in them, we have no reason to conclude that they will ever cease to be what they now are . . .
Assuming then, my postulata as granted I say, that the power of population is indefinitely greater than the power in the earth to produce subsistence for man.

---

1. William and Paul Paddock, *FAMINE—1975!* (Boston: Little, Brown, 1967).

Population when unchecked, increases in a geometrical ratio. Subsistence increases only in an arithmetical ratio. A slight acquaintance with numbers will show the immensity of the first power in comparison of the second.

By that law of our nature which makes food necessary to the life of man, the effects of these two unequal powers must be kept equal.

There are those who will argue that Malthusian theory is no longer functional—that science and technology are fully capable of solving man's subsistence problem by new methods of farming and synthetic foods. The arguments seem to have their foundation in a "blind faith" in science and technology; however, the age of innocent faith in science and technology is being challenged and appears to be nearing an end.

The Population Problem—A Perspective

In 1830 there were 1 billion people on the face of the earth. By 1930 the number had risen to 2 billion and by 1960 there were 3 billion. At present the world population is approximately 3.5 billion persons.

It took from the beginning of time to 1830 to produce the first billion people; it took a century (1830-1930) to produce the next billion; the third billion appeared in a mere 30 years (1930-60) and it is projected that the fourth billion will be with us by 1975.

The United States and Canada with a population of nearly 215 million and a growth rate of 1.6 percent a year will, if the present growth rate continues to the year 2000, show a population increase of 80 percent. This will result in a total population growth for the U.S. and Canada of 173 million persons in a relatively short period of time.

Modern man has had a tendency to view population growth as a problem only in underdeveloped countries, such as China and India. He has failed to realize that at the present rate of growth (1.6 percent) the size of the United States population will in less than a century exceed the size of the present population of China, which has a considerably larger land mass.

In the developing nations of the world population is growing at a most rapid rate. With birth rates remaining high and death rates dropping sharply, many countries of Latin America, Asia and Africa now grow ten times as fast as they did a century ago. At the present growth rates many will double and some may even triple their present population before the year 2000.

The development of these nations is actually being challenged in some cases by the rapid population increase. The good economic development they may have experienced has failed to keep pace with the population increases resulting in a worsened quality of living. Actually, this overbalance of population growth threatens the success of many of these countries in their attempts to rid themselves of the problems of poverty, hunger, disease, overcrowding and illiteracy. For many it is a desperate and depressing situation.

Factors Influencing the Population Explosion

Traditionally population has been controlled by famine and disease. Disease has usually been the actual limiting factor. Thanks to rapid advances in medical sciences disease has been sharply curtailed as an effective controller of population growth. Medical science and improved living conditions have also contributed to the population problem by increasing the life span of man. In the United States in 1850 the average human life span was 40 years; in 1900 it was 49 years and presently it stands at 70 years. Man in the U. S. today is spending almost twice as much time on the face of the earth as did his ancestors of a century ago.

In some countries of the world the longevity figures are even higher. In Sweden, Norway and the Netherlands the average life span is approximately 72 years. India on the other hand shows the lowest—46 years.

A growing imbalance between birth rates and death rates is responsible for the current rapid population growth. With death rates still declining and birth rates persisting, the overpopulation problem can only worsen. Just look at the following actual example of man's own reproductive potential, so little realized by the average person.

John Eli Miller, an Ohio farmer, has the opportunity of witnessing the reproductive potential of man in his own life time, within his own family. At the time of his death at age 95, he was survived by 5 of his 7 children, 61 grandchildren, 338 great grandchildren and 6 great-great grandchildren, a total of 410 *living* descendents. Mr. Miller provides us with 410 living examples of the high reproductive potential of man. Admittedly an extreme example, this points up a potential threat that could very well prove disastrous.

A look at the birth rate statistics in the United States gives evidence of early marriages as another possible contributing factor to the population problem. Early marriages appear to be on the increase in the United States. Recent figures show that in over 50 percent of the marriages in the United States the female partner was under the age of twenty. This age group in turn also accounts for the highest birth rate among married females. In the United States in 1960 the birth rate among married women under the age of 20 was 54 children per 100 women. Married women between the ages of 20-24 showed a birth rate of 35 children per 100 women. In the 25-29 age group the figure dropped to 22 births per 100. Of the illegitimate births, 40 percent were by women under the age of 20. This is in relation to the 240,200 total recorded illegitimate births in the U. S. in 1961.

Religious ideologies and cultural factors have also been shown to be factors contributing to the rapid population growth in some areas of the world.

Looking into the future and viewing the problem on a global scale, one sees an even more complicated dilemma. It is being predicted that medical advances will continue to prolong man's life span. By the turn of the century research could reach a point where sugar can be created from water and carbon dioxide. The biological revolution is fully upon us, and the effects of its achievements may mean a further increase in human population coinciding with a time when the world could least afford it.

It appears that world society is constantly being faced with an ever-growing number of situations where "good means" can result in catastrophic ends, as evidenced by the aforementioned advances in medical science and technology ushering in the present environmental crisis.

Proposed Solutions to the Problem of Population

The solution to the problem is a complex one. The Panel of the United Nations Association stated that the high rates of population growth "impair individual rights, jeopardize national goals and threaten international stability." While this is true, the problems inherent in population control measures may also serve to "impair human rights, jeopardize national goals and threaten international stability." Unquestionably "individual rights" are a matter of paramount concern in any program of population control. It is also evident, when considering measures for population control, that such factors as religious dogma, societal values, economic and cultural backgrounds are all relevant to national goals, and to international stability when on a global basis.

For full comprehension of the problems inherent in setting up any proposed method of population control certain basic questions must be asked and the answers attempted: What is meant by control? Who is to do the controlling? Toward what contemplated goals are the controls being planned?

Suggested methods for population control are to be found at every turn. They run the gamut, from changing existing tax laws so as to discourage rather than encourage reproductiveness—to the restrictive "issuance of coupons" entitling couples to produce children. Some view legalized abortion as presently being employed in Japan as a partial solution to the population problem. Family Planning Clinics have been in existence for some time in a number of countries and have had some success in reducing birth rates. In some of the underdeveloped countries, government programs have been established for the purpose of providing free instruction and materials for birth control to massive segments of the population. Some of these programs have even offered "monetary rewards" in an attempt to get the population involved with the program.

All proposed solutions to the problem, and they are many, have encountered major obstacles such as lack of public support, feasibility, human ethics, cultural factors, etc. None are programmed on a massive public scale to help the individual reach a "control" decision based on his responsibilities to himself, his potential family and society.

There is little question that in the more advanced societies the possibilities for successful solution are greater, resting as they do with the "educated" individual who has the ability to interact with his environment in intelligent and humane ways.

The solution in the underdeveloped countries is more difficult. Education and educational systems are in some cases virtually nonexistent and the illiteracy rate consequently high, the cultural taboos many. The combination presents a real challenge to a world attempting to control its population growth.

In a message to the Ninety-first Congress, on July 18, 1969, President Nixon, in calling for the establishment of a Commission on Population Growth and the American Future, stated:

> One of the most serious challenges to human dignity in the last third of this century will be the growth of the population. Whether man's response to that challenge will be a cause for pride or for despair in the year 2000 will depend very much on what we do today. If we now begin our work in an appropriate manner, and if we continue to devote a considerable amount of attention and energy to this problem then mankind will be able to surmount this challenge as it has surmounted so many during the long march of civilization.
>
> When future generations evaluate the record of our time, one of the most important factors in their judgment will be in the way in which we responded to population growth.

Man can meet the challenge. Man must meet the challenge. The technology is available. Research on methods of contraception has produced a number of very effective methods of birth control from the intra-uterine device to the oral contraceptive. It is apparent that in the near future mankind will be able to control the "fertility process" simply by administering a single injection into a immature female that will render her incapable of fertility until an antidote is given. This, however, would be no solution, since the problem is a human one, and needs to be solved in humane manner. The success of any humane program of population control rests clearly within the realm of human values, attitudes and behavior.

If man is truly concerned about controlling population he must deal directly with these attitudes and values of the individuals concerned. The sum total of all scientific advances in contraceptive methodology is worth little if by reason of attitudes, human values, and behavior the individuals concerned do not choose to make use of any of them.

Today's population control concept calls for the new ethic of the two-child family to replace what appears to be the American dream of three or more children. While some ask for legislative measures that would place severe restrictions on the number of children a couple could have, the realistic and humane solution lies in a reorientation, perhaps drastic, of the individual's philosophy pertinent to his reproductive responsibility. Should man choose not to solve the population problem by humane standards, nature will solve it her way, be it through pollution, pestilence, disease or mass starvation. The real hope is in the development in man of an ecological conscience based on the prime value of humanness and the quality of life. It is in relation to human worth and human values that the decisions regarding population must ultimately be made.

Suggestions for Individual Action

- Limit the size of your family to no more than two children. If a larger family is desired consider the adoption of additional children.
- Support educational ventures such as Planned Parenthood in an effort to educate the general public relative to the population problem and birth control methods.
- Use every opportunity to point out that pollution problems in general are directly related to overpopulation.

1. Develop a brief (footnoted) paper outlining the major factors contributory to the population explosion.
2. Read a book (see bibliography) or article in a professional journal dealing with the population problem and give your personal reaction to the material presented in a short paper.
3. Much has been written relative to the possible role of liberalized abortion measures in helping curb population growth. Search out one such article and react to it in a short paper.
4. Read the piece by Thomas Robert Malthus, "An Essay on the Principle of Population," written in 1798 and react to the theory presented on the basis of the current world population situation. Is his theory at all applicable to the present dilemma?

CHAPTER 4

Air Pollution
and Man

*Our choices are narrow. We can remain
indoors and live like moles for an unspeci-
fied number of days each year. We can
issue gas masks to a large segment of the
population. We can live in domed cities.
Or we can take action to stop fouling the
air we breath.*

—JOHN W. GARDNER

The basic use of the atmosphere is to sustain life. The environment
is an ocean of air, of which each man must inhale approximately 450
cubic feet daily in order to obtain the necessary oxygen. The quality of
this air must be such that it does not foul the gas exchange mechanisms
for even a short time. While man can go months without food, days
without water, he can only remain alive for a few minutes without sufficient oxygen.

Yet man has polluted this air—in some cases to a very critical level.
Tokyo policemen must return regularly to headquarters for a period of
oxygen inhalation: in that same city vending machines in arcades and
coffee shops make oxygen readily available to the man on the street.
Today, on this planet Earth, man is buying a whiff of oxygen and taking
an essential "on-the-job oxygen break." It seems utterly incomprehensible
that man can concern himself with providing air for man on the moon,
while at the same time so fouling the air here on earth.

The degree to which man has fouled his air is startling. In the
United States alone it is estimated that more than 110,000 deaths each
year are due in part to air pollution. Air pollution has been responsible
for a number of incidents of massive death. In one siege alone (1952)
four thousand Londoners died. In 1956, in a mere eighteen-hour period,
one thousand persons died in New York City as a result of a heavy
smog that settled over the city. The list of such incidents has grown to
outrageous proportions.

No Real Boundaries

Among the major problems relative to air pollution is its complete lack of respect for boundaries. A recent newspaper headline reads "Pollution Defies Europe's Borders," and the story that followed explained the resultant danger to fresh water fish and forests in Oslo, Norway. This danger is the result of the rising acidity of rain and snow, attributable to wastes from as far away as Britain and possibly West Germany.[2]

Eruptions of volcanos at the turn of the century gave evidence of how the air could become polluted on a planet-wide basis from only one source. For more than two years after each eruption of the Alaskan Volcano Mount Katmai (1900) clouds of fine volcanic dust blanketed the sky throughout the world.

The Origin of the Atmosphere

In order to fully understand the implications of air pollution, it is first necessary to examine the evolution and functions of the air that envelops the earth. This more than seven-mile-high expanse of atmosphere serves to intercept the sun's deadly short-wave radiation. It destroys invading meteorites, insulates the earth's surface and distributes heat. It provides the setting for the earth's weather and the air necessary for both physical and life processes on the planet.

The original atmosphere (3-5 billion years ago) was composed of a large variety of gases. Conditions were extremely hot and gas molecules picked up enough speed to burst free of the atmosphere. This is presumably what happened to the earth's original atmosphere. These layers of gas had served as an insulating blanket, and with their departure heat gradually radiated from the planet. The cooling surface squeezed in on the warmer core creating enormous internal pressures causing volcanic craters to burst forth. During the era of volcanic eruptions many gases that had been trapped in the earth's core were discharged. Since the surface temperature surrounding the earth had dropped the gases did not escape and remained to evolve into our present atmosphere.

The evolution of this atmosphere provided the initial gases that supported simple life and from that point on all evolution patterns followed—effected by environmental interactions that regulated what survived and what failed to survive. Supporting cycles developed and within such a framework evolved man, the gaseous atmosphere and all other environmental factors. Thus man evolved in a sense as a "natural part" of the environment, not in conflict with it, but rather as an integral part of it.

---

2. *New York Times*, 11 January, 1970, sec. I., p. 24.

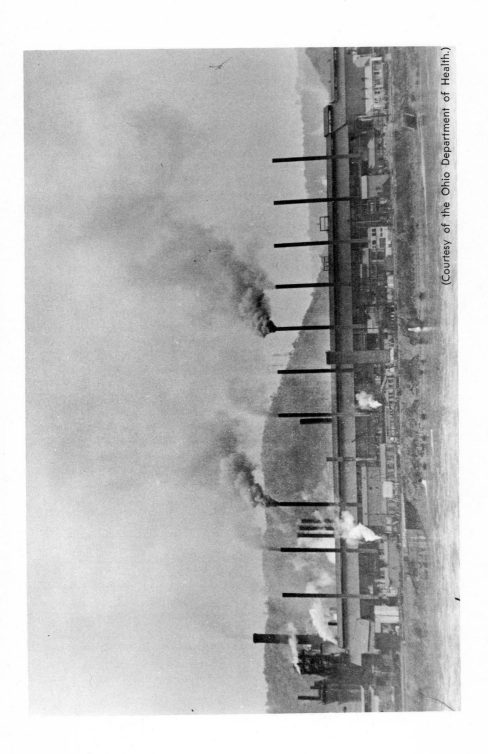

(Courtesy of the Ohio Department of Health.)

The Present Atmosphere

The earth's surface is immersed in a gaseous atmosphere the composition of which varies with the altitude. We will, however, concern ourselves only with the composition of the air at earth's surface. Pure, dry air contains by volume 20.92 percent oxygen, 78.14 percent nitrogen, 0.04 percent carbon dioxide and .09 percent argon and trace elements of other gases. Water vapor may be present in natural air up to the saturation point. All other substances in the air, whether gases, vapors, or solid particles, must be considered contaminates. These contaminates fall into two general types, natural and man-made. Natural pollutants consist of pollen, spores and natural dust. Man-made pollutants result from man's many activities—from simple breathing to giant industrial processes.

Contamination of the Air

Many factors are responsible for contamination of the air. The population explosion, the growing affluence and resultant increase in consumption, expanding technology and other factors have intermingled to present man with the very complex dilemma of attempting to determine who and what are responsible for this contamination. It is not feasible, even if it were possible, to cover all the sources and types of pollutants. It *must* be borne in mind, however, that *all* sources of pollution, whether large or small, contribute to the total air pollution problem.

CHART I

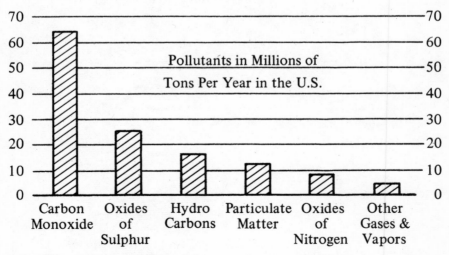

Source: U. S. Department of Health, Education, and Welfare, Public Health Service. Proceedings: The National Conference on Air Pollution. Washington, D. C., 1966, p. 333.

CHART II

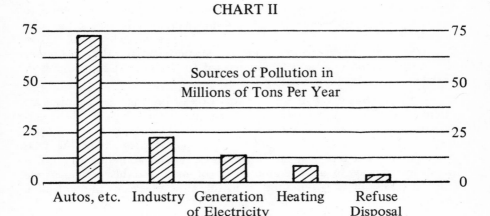

Source: U. S. Department of Health, Education, and Welfare, Public Health Service. Proceedings: The National Conference on Air Pollution. Washington, D. C., 1966. p. 447.

The Natural Pollutants

Pollen Grains. Spores and pollen given off by flowers and fungi have proven to be a real menace to persons who are allergic to them. Surveys have shown that as much as ten to fifteen percent of the general public in some areas of the nation are allergic to ragweed pollen alone. This allergy results in what is commonly known as hayfever. While appearing to be a minor disorder, hayfever can develop into chronic asthma and so become a significant cause of death. So important an ailment is it that public health departments across the country operate ragweed monitoring stations to furnish ragweed pollen counts during the pollination season. Radio stations may be heard broadcasting the results of these daily counts which indicate the amount of concentration of ragweed pollen present in the air during a given 24-hour period.

These pollen grains, a form of aeroallergies, are very small, and serve as antigens in an antigen-antibody (allergic) reaction when they settle in the nasal passages of persons sensitive to them. A daily count of "7" or more is indicative of a pollen concentration sufficiently high that those who are allergic are apt to notice hayfever symptoms. These counts serve as a warning to hayfever sufferers to take the necessary precautionary measures, such as to stay indoors and to use air-conditioners. They are also indicators as to the "severity" of the hayfever season for the physician.

Dust Particles. Dust particles, particularly if they are 1/25,000 of an inch in size or smaller, present a very real air pollution problem. Sources of such particles are high winds, earthquakes, volcanic eruptions and traffic. Particles this small, regardless of the source, tend to become permanent residents in the atmosphere, while larger particles usually fall to the ground near their source. Since particles smaller than 1/25,000 of an inch in size frequent the air one breathes they also enter the lungs and become a potential hazard to the critical functioning of the delicate pulmonary tissues.

Carbon Dioxide. Carbon dioxide excess presents a complex air pollution problem. We know that nearly all living things produce carbon dioxide as a waste product and that it is also a by-product of combustion. Green plants are responsible for removing much of the CO_2 from the air and replacing it with oxygen. As the abundance of green plants gives way to an overabundance of man and his activities, we find an excess of CO_2 building up in the atmosphere, to the sum of 6 million tons a year.

Definite evidence proves that the concentration of carbon dioxide in the atmosphere as a whole has increased about ten percent during this century, from approximately 290 parts per million (ppm) in 1900 to over 320 parts per million at present.[3] While there is no direct toxic effect on humans from an increase of carbon dioxide (provided the available oxygen is not greatly reduced) there is an indirect adverse effect warranting considerable attention.

CO_2 and the "Greenhouse Effect." The increase in the atmosphere's carbon dioxide level has been accompanied by a corresponding increase in the temperature of the atmosphere. The temperature of an average U. S. winter has climbed 3 1/2 degrees in the past sixty years. What we know as the "greenhouse effect" puts the overall picture in better perspective and helps to explain this rise in the earth's temperature (see figure 2).

Since CO_2 is one of the principle substances in the air which absorb and emit infrared radiation and as such is responsible for the "greenhouse effect" there is much concern about its concentration. Assuming the figures to be correct, it is quite possible that the average temperature of the earth could rise forty degrees (F.) within 400 years—unless changes are brought about in the concentrations of CO_2.

Continuation of this temperature rise could result in the melting of the ice caps over Greenland and Antarctica and cause a rise of sea level and flooding of populated coastal areas such as New York, Boston, Los Angeles. A report of the President's Science Advisory Committee stated: "The melting of the Arctic ice cap would raise sea level by 400

3. U. S. Department of Health, Education and Welfare, Public Health Service. *Proccedings: The National Conference on Air Pollution.* Washington, D. C., 1966, p. 447.

Radiant Energy from Sun   Radiant Energy from Sun

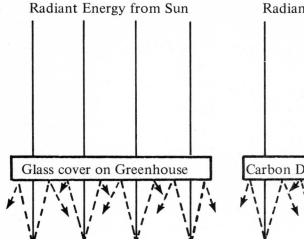

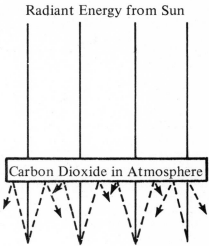

Energy trapped in the form of heat, which cannot escape from the glass shield. Thus the warmth of a green-house, even in winter.

Energy trapped in the form of heat—which, due to the increased CO_2 acting as a glass shield, cannot escape as efficiently as before. Thus the greater the CO_2 concentration the more heat trapped.

feet. If 1,000 years were required to melt the ice cap, the sea level would rise about four feet every 10 years, 40 feet per century."[4]

Another theory however, has been advanced, that runs contrary to the "greenhouse effect" explanation. It is based on the evidence that particulate matter in the atmosphere is increasing in concentration. These particles have the effect of forming a shield-like barrier in the atmosphere that would tend to limit the penetration of the sun's radiant energy and thus bringing about a cooling effect on the planet—and perhaps ultimately another ice age. There is presently considerable controversy regarding the validity of this theory. It does, however, serve to point up the extent to which man has contaminated the environment and in the problems inherent in such uncontrolled contamination.

CO_2 and the Physiology of Living Organisms. Another problem related to the increased amount of CO_2 in the air deals more directly with the physiology of living organisms. As stated earlier, carbon dioxide and oxygen are involved in a cyclic process that includes the green plants and nearly all animal forms. Considering the earth as a closed ecological

4. President's Science Advisory Committee, *Restoring the Quality of Our Environment* (Washington, D. C.: Government Printing Office, 1965).

system and understanding fully the real significance of this cyclic process, one cannot help but be concerned about the rapidly diminishing number of green plants on the face of the earth coinciding with the phenomenally increasing number of humans. Presently the plants of the world in a single year are responsible for the production of nearly 400 billion tons of O_2, while consuming nearly 500 billion tons of CO_2.

It does not take much of a scientific mind to see that man's very survival as an oxygen-breathing organism is being placed in jeopardy as one of his main sources of oxygen yields to the "saws" of progress and development. This, coupled with the fact that these green plants are also a major factor in the necessary absorption of carbon dioxide, and the full magnitude of the dilemma posed by the disruption of this life-preservation cycle becomes evident.

Man–Made Pollutants

Man has very ingeniously developed a large variety of air pollutant sources. They range in type from the giant industrial stacks that release their gaseous wastes well up into the atmosphere to that very "personal portable air polluter," commonly known as the cigarette.

Pollutants from Gasoline-Powered Vehicles. The more than 100 million gasoline-powered vehicles presently jamming U. S. highways are responsible for a variety of air pollutants. These pollutants are principally hydrocarbons and other organic compounds, carbon monoxide, nitrogen oxides, hydrogen, and lead compounds.

Studies have shown that *one thousand* operating automobiles contribute approximately the following amounts of these pollutants to the atmosphere per day:

Carbon monoxide	3.2 tons
Hydrocarbons (organic vapors)	400-800 pounds
Nitrous Oxides	100-200 pounds

Hydrocarbons—The auto is the principle contributor to hydrocarbon emissions. Hydrocarbons are compounds of carbon and hydrogen that react with oxide of nitrogen in sunlight to form photochemical smog. This particular type of pollution has gained much ill fame in the Los Angeles basin. The "end-product-mixture" is damaging to plants, causes irritation to the eyes and mucous membranes of humans, and reduces visibility.

Carbon Monoxide—The principal contaminate from autos, by weight, is carbon monoxide. Its concentration in the atmosphere presents a very real threat to human life, especially in urban areas. The toxic effects of carbon monoxide (due to its affinity with hemoglobin) have long been known. Carbon monoxide begins to be hazardous to humans at a concentration of about 100 ppm. if the level is maintained for several hours. That level is within reach at present in areas where automobile traffic is excessively heavy.

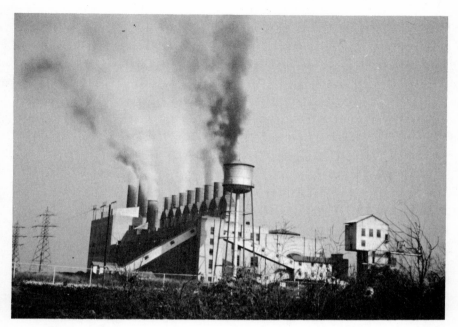

Man's capability to "foul" his environment has increased with the rapid advances in technology, and the growth of population. More population requires more electricity, which results in more pollution . . . a vicious cycle that challenges man's very survival. (Courtesy of the Ohio Department of Health.)

The Auto and the Combustion Problem. Most automotive emission, about 85 percent, originates from the combustion process (vapors from evaporating fuel account for the other 15 percent). Carbon monoxide and small amounts of unburned hydrocarbons are given off because combustion of the fuel-air mixture in the engine is not complete. If all our driving was at steady speeds on open highways exhaust emissions would be no problem. The exhaust difficulty arises when an engine is idling as constantly occurs in city driving. In such circumstances the proper mixture for complete combustion is not rich enough to keep a car running smoothly. The mixture changes to meet the needs of different engine speeds and at low speeds the overall emission quantity increases. Thus, city driving produces much more exhaust pollutants than does driving on the open highway.

It must be kept in mind that while the emissions from a single car are relatively small, the number of cars is not—100 million motor vehicles currently on the highways being responsible for 60 percent of all U. S. air pollution! As a result of this combination of figures the auto makers have been hit by Federal legislation for a "clean car" by 1975.

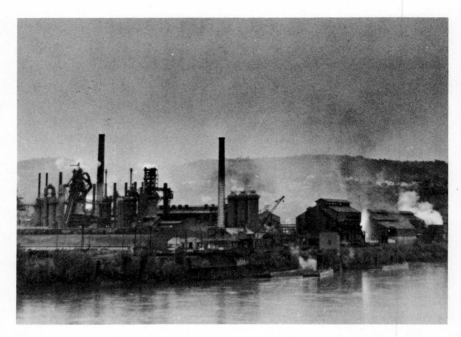

Pollution concentrations increase as a haze hangs over the community. In some areas these concentrations have reached a critically dangerous level. (Courtesy of the Ohio Department of Health.)

The Thermal Inversion

An atmospheric condition known as thermal inversion has served to compound the air pollution problem in certain sections of the country.

The temperature of the atmosphere normally decreases about five degrees (F.) with each 1,000 feet of elevation. During the day, the radiant energy of the sun warms the earth's surface, which in turn warms the layer of air directly adjacent to it. This warmer air is less dense than the cooler air above and rises through this cooler air mass. This warm rising air carries with it most of the contaminates it has received from the earth's environment and is replaced by a cooler, more dense and less contaminated air, which warms and in turn follows this same pattern.

In a valley and under certain other conditions this process can go askew. When atmospheric conditions permit a cold air mass to form under a warmer air mass, a thermal inversion is formed. Under these circumstances the pollutants given off continue to build up in this lower air mass, which remains trapped by the inversion system. Since this air does not move out, and may stay for a prolonged period of time, the quality of this air mass deteriorates and becomes a real hazard to health.

Pollutants continue to collect and become concentrated in the air space near the ground (in some cases this air mass may only be thirty feet high) until the warm air rises high enough to permit the cooler air to escape and the inversion to break. Winds may also serve to break up a thermal inversion.

Human Health and Air Pollution

At a recent medical research conference sponsored by the American Medical Association it was pointed out that air pollution may be contributing to diseases of the stomach, heart and respiratory system. The researchers found that cancer deaths in the highest risk group, ages fifty to sixty-nine, were almost doubled in areas with large amounts of suspended particles of soot and ash in the air.[5] Chemical pollutants in the air have been found to be closely linked with such diseases as hypertensive heart disease, cardiovascular disease, pneumonia, lung cancer, chronic bronchitis and emphysema.

The problem of air pollution is an obvious one. Man needs only to examine his immediate surroundings to recognize his constant exposure to pollutants. A mere whiff of air in many parts of the country provides ample evidence of their presence. Driving into some of the metropolitan areas one is struck by the continuous cover of haze that blankets the city, even on a cloudless day. Exposure to smoke pollutants is very evident in the many public facilities such as buses, airplanes, restaurants, and classrooms, where smoking is allowed. It is a very real problem, presenting even in these simple situations an ethical dilemma, where the "individual right" to smoke and pollute clashes with the "public right" to breathe clean air.

Man will have to solve this dilemma if he is to live in symbiotic harmony with his fellow man, and in the environment at large at well.

Suggestions for Individual Action

- When purchasing an automobile consider the horsepower of the engine, size of the body and effectiveness of pollution abatement devices. A large car requires more horsepower to move and as a result generally produces more pollutants than a smaller, less powerful one.
- Walk, bicycle or use rapid transport rather than your own car whenever possible. The formation of car pools is an effective method of reducing automobile-caused pollution.

---

5. "Research Strengthens Link Between Air Pollution and Disease," *Today's Health* 47 (January 1969): 1.

- Avoid any type of open-air burning. Do not burn leaves or trash. Build up a compose pile, which will provide excellent fertilizer for plants and shrubs by returning the nutrients to the soil.
- Stop smoking. You are not only polluting your own lungs— you are also polluting the lungs of those around you.
- Report any suspected sources of pollution to the proper authorities. Be a "voice to save the environment" on a local level. Speak out against such practices as open and controlled dump burning, etc.
- Select clean burning fuels such as natural gas, whenever possible, instead of coal, oil or gasoline.

1. Develop a paper converging on population and pollution as related problems. In doing so, touch upon the following major points:
   a. Give evidence as to the source and magnitude of the problem.
   b. Discuss proposed solutions to the problem and give your reaction to the one you consider most feasible.
2. Develop a listing of all visible sources of air pollution in your community. Include such information as source, type and location of the pollution. You may see fit to supplement such information with a map pin-pointing community pollution sources.
3. Contact the air-monitoring division of your local health department for the purpose of investigating the measures (such as air monitoring procedures) being taken to protect the community from air pollution hazards.
4. Read a book (see bibliography) or article in a professional journal dealing with the air pollution problem and react to the material presented from a personal point of view.

CHAPTER 5

Water Pollution
and Man

*Till taught by pain, men really knows not
what good water's worth.*

—Lord Byron

Water is the great supporter of life. The first inhabitants of the earth were conceived in water. Man still gives evidence of this close relationship and dependence on the sea from which he came. The blood in his veins is as salty as the sea in which he was conceived. Eighty-five percent of man's brain tissue is water. The human fetus undergoes development while submerged in a liquid and water continues to be the prime medium and ingredient for the many chemical activities carried out in the human system.

Man, in his search for possible life forms on another planet, has focused attention on the presence of water as a basic indicator of the potential for such life.

Sources of Water

Pure water is tasteless, colorless and odorless. Water in "pure" form, however, is a rare occurrence in nature, as it always contains some sort of impurities. Even rain water picks up dust, smoke, fumes and gases as it precipitates from the atmosphere. It may also pick up air-borne bacteria, spores and pollen.

Sources of water may be classified into three major areas.
1. Rain water.
2. Surface water (as found in ponds, lakes, streams and reservoirs).
3. Ground water (from wells, both shallow and deep, and springs).

Water in the Environment

A body of water is a dynamic system, constantly receiving a wide range of liquids, gases and solids. Natural waters provide a habitat for

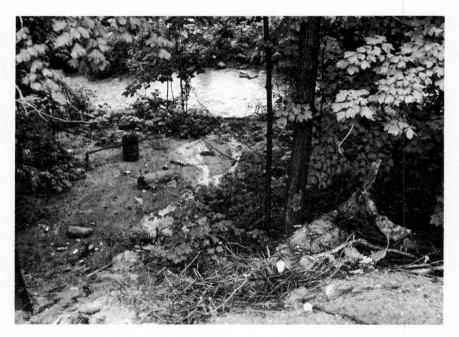

What was once a lovely picnic site has been destroyed by man's lack of concern for his environment. While it once served for man's enjoyment, this site is now a threat to his well-being. (Photo by J. Phillips.)

many organisms—single microorganisms to complex plant and animal life. Water is of itself essential to the support of both plant and animal life. It is one of the most precious compounds on the planet Earth. Yet man has, through his unceasing activities and processes, over-polluted much of his available water supply. Water may be considered polluted when it is unsuitable for its intended purpose or use: municipal water supply, recreation, industry or in support of plant or animal life. Water may be rendered unsuitable or polluted when it becomes over-burdened with any of the following:

1. Infectious disease-producing agents.
2. Organic wastes of human and animal origin.
3. Plant nutrients.
4. Inorganic chemicals.
5. Organic chemicals.
6. Sediments.
7. Radiation.
8. Thermal factors (a change in temperature).
9. Hard surface run-off.

Polluted Rivers

Man has begun to witness some alarming examples of the pollution of his vital water supply. As a case in point, in the summer of 1969 the Cuyahoga river in northern Ohio caught fire! There was no immediate disaster to account for the fire, no oil barge that burst open. The river's water was so contaminated from man's daily activities that it became a hazard by virtue of its very existence. A fire alarm turned in on a river, the Cuyahoga River, U. S. A., on a warm summer's day in 1969 . . . truly an event to remember!

As an indicator of the vivid reality and the broad extent of the water pollution problem consider the many rivers (in addition to the Cuyahoga) that have gained undesirable recognition by being the most polluted in the nation. They are: the Ohio, the Houston Ship Canal, the Rouge (Michigan), the Buffalo, the Passaic and the Arthurhill (New Jersey), the Merrimack (between New Hampshire and Massachusetts), the Androscoggin (Maine), and the Escambia in Florida. These rivers have been polluted by a variety of man-made toxins which include oil, municipal sewage, mine and manufacturing acids.

Nor has man stopped with the rivers. One of the more vivid examples is Lake Erie, now become a dead body of water! In addition to sewage it receives an estimated ton of chemicals a minute from industrial plants in four states.

In terms of collective parameters, the leading source of controllable man-made water pollutants in the United States is manufacturing, with domestic wastes second.[6]

Other sources include urban and agricultural livestock feedlot runoff, acid mine drainage, and watercraft.

Water Pollutants from Agriculture

Water pollutants from agricultural processes present a major control problem, due to the multiplicity of factors involved. The major water pollutants from agriculture are:
1. Sediment from the erosion of cropland.
2. Animal wastes.
3. Pesticides.
4. Compounds of phosphorous and nitrogen that have their origin in chemical fertilizers.

Also of major concern is the rapidly growing animal feeding industry. Cattle are presently being raised in feeding lots that allow only 500

---

6. American Chemical Society, *Cleaning Our Environment: The Chemical Basis for Action* (Washington, D. C., 1969), p. 96.

square feet per animal. This method of raising cattle has proven to be more efficient and profitable than the "open range" method. The wastes of the cattle are thus concentrated in a small area, making for a very noxious condition and presenting a real problem in waste disposal. Locating these feeding pens on the side of a hill for "wash off" effects has compounded the problem. A feedlot with 10,000 head of cattle gives off wastes equivalent to those of a city of 45,000. The overall waste produced by farm animals in the U. S. has been estimated to total about twenty times that of human population. It is clearly evident that one of the prime factors in water pollution centers around run-off from areas contaminated by livestock and poultry wastes, particularly cattle feedlots.

Domestic Wastes

Domestic wastes are a major contributor to the water pollution problem, second only to wastes from manufacturing processes. A typical city of 100,000 persons produces the following wastes every day of the year.
- One ton of detergents
- Seventeen tons of organic suspended particles
- Sixteen tons of organic dissolved solids
- Eight tons of inorganic dissolved solids

The problem this creates is compounded by the fact that some of the cities and towns that have sewage disposal plants still discharge untreated wastes into rivers and streams.

An inventory of muncipal sewage treatment plants in the United States during the 1960s showed some 118 million people living in communities served by sewer systems. Yet about 20 percent of the waste water remained untreated, 28 percent received only primary treatment and 52 percent received some kind of secondary treatment.[7] Since these figures have been gathered some improvements have been made, but much remains to be done.

While most cities have sewage disposal systems, many smaller communities do not. These smaller communities use septic tanks and cesspools to dispose of the bulk of their sewage wastes. Since this method of disposal depends on bacterial action that decomposes the sewage and then filters it through seepage beds as it returns it to the soil, it has presented a water pollution problem, particularly in areas of high population density.

In cases where the septic tanks are not properly cared for, the bacteria may be killed off and the wastes do not decompose. Detergents have been a factor in the destruction of the bacteria. Houses that

7. *American Chemical Society, Cleaning Our Environment*, p. 108.

are located close together, and depend on individual septic tanks and seepage beds to handle their waste, have in some cases saturated the ground with sewage. This is particularly true in developments having homes located close together on very small lots.

The danger to the water supply is evident, particularly if these same homes are deriving their water from wells since wastes that are not properly decomposed find their way into these wells, or seep into streams, or even in some cases penetrate downward toward a water table or underground stream from which the wells may be fed. For this primary reason (there are others) anyone that has a home disposing of its wastes through a septic tank or cesspool must carry out the maintenance necessary for such a system. Information on the topic is generally available through local health department offices.

Municipal wastes, by contrast, undergo treatment through a sewage treatment plant, in two stages:

1. Primary treatment, where grit removal, screening, grinding flocculation and sedimentation take place.
2. Secondary treatment, where bio-oxidation takes place using such processes as trickling filter and activated sludge.

After thorough treatment these wastes are returned to the environment and reenter various natural cycles.

The Process of Eutrophication

Lake Tahoe, partly in Nevada and partly in California, has drawn much attention, both as a vacation paradise and as potential ecological disaster.

The gambling casinos on the lake's edge, handling tens of thousands of guests, have been cited for emptying their sewage into this crystal clear lake. Two hundred tons of sewage a day, it is estimated, enter Lake Tahoe. In addition, the land has been exposed to erosion due to the fact that standing timber around the lake has been cut in the development process. The nutrients that normally would remain in the soil have been washed into the lake and as a result the algae and other plant life are being "over fed."

These two factors, the inordinate increases of nutrients from the sewage wastes and of the minerals (primarily nitrogen and phosphorous) washed in from the exposed hillsides, result in a rapid acceleration of the process of eutrophication—the natural aging process that occurs in still or nearly still bodies of water. Normally over a period of many years these bodies of water undergo a change and "fill in" as plant growth in them flourishes, dies and decomposes, depleting available oxygen (the decay of dead matter involves the process of oxidation).

This depletion of oxygen and the accumulation of the decayed plant sludge alters the aquatic life forms and a swamp condition develops. This in turn dries out and becomes a land mass. The process normally

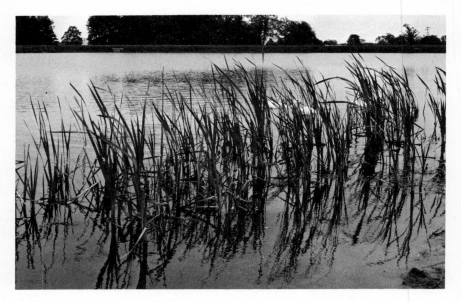

Over a period of many years, bodies of still or nearly still water undergo a natural aging process that causes them to "fill in" as plant growth in them flourishes, dies and decomposes. (Photo by J. Phillips.)

takes thousands of years, but when an overabundance of nutrients becomes available to the algae and other plant life in a body of water, the aging process is greatly speeded up.

As a result of the increased rate of eutrophication in Lake Tahoe, there is much concern about the future of this crystal clear lake. Measures can be taken to save the lake but these measures would have been unnecessary if an ecological consciousness had prevailed when the resort area was undergoing development.

Rapid eutrophication of bodies of water has been witnessed in many parts of the country. The run-off of fertilizers applied to farm lands and the use of household detergents have also contributed to this problem. These agricultural fertilizers and detergents have one major chemical compound in common—phosphates, which eventually find their way into waterways and add to the problems of rapid eutrophication. The problem has reached so high a level that it has caused the Federal Water Pollution Control Administration to urge legislation restricting the production of phosphates in detergents.

Other Factors Have Contributed to the Problem

Man has, through his lack of ecological perspective, managed to foul the waters in a variety of ways.

In choosing sites to build homes quickly, developers went to the valleys and meadows, without considering their proximity to underground water supplies that could easily be fouled by an overabundance of housing. Ecological studies, undertaken before developing started, could have prevented this problem. Hawaii is the only state in the nation that is attempting to solve this and similar environmental problems by "state zoned lands."

Dams are known to ruin a river as a free flowing stream. It is evident that many dams not only are of temporary value (many are filling in) but they have also been responsible for many ecological side effects.

Twelve miles off the Long Island shore, out in the Atlantic, lies a twenty square mile "dead sea." It has been made by man, the result of a number of his own actions. Metropolitan New York sewage plants have been dumping sewage sludge and dredging spoils in this location for forty years. Restrictions have been imposed by the Food and Drug Administration that prohibits the harvesting of shell fish within a six-mile limit of this dead sea.

Nuclear Power Plants. Nuclear power plants are becoming increasingly evident as the need for electricity soars upward. Yet they too have provided man with another dilemma relative to his environment. In the boiling-water type of nuclear power plant, the heat of the reactor, upon contact with water, converts it to steam which in turn drives the turbine generators to produce electricity. Since water is so obviously vital to this process, these plants have been located adjacent to rivers or other large bodies of water. Water for the process is taken from these bodies of water and returned at a much higher temperature. It may, besides, contain small amounts of radioactive wastes. Here man is presented with the dual problems of thermal pollution and radioactive waste disposal. The state of Minnesota has made it a requirement that all water used for such processes must be returned at the same temperature it was taken.

Marine Pollution. Marine pollution presents man with perhaps his most complex water dilemma. It even effects the very air he breathes. Man's major source of oxygen is the plankton, the microscopic plant life of the seas. Plankton serves not only as a major oxygen source but absorbs large quantities of carbon dioxide. If man fouls the environment of these microscopic plants he may also foul the air he breathes. Which is the greater problem, air pollution or water pollution—or can they even be separated?

The oceans of the world are being polluted a variety of ways. They have served as dumping grounds for many of the wastes of man. The rivers that empty into these great bodies of water carry in them a great variety and quantity of wastes.

Oil drilling on the continental shelf and the transportation of oil have both added a new dimension to the problem. The Torry Canyon, a tanker whose wreckage poured forth 100,000 tons of oil that fouled the beaches of France and Britain, provided the first incident of real concern. The problem has grown in potential as the tankers have gotten large and larger; first 30,000 tons, then 100,000 tons, 250,000 tons and now 800,000 ton capacities. Offshore oil drilling rigs have also contributed to the problem. Recently, an oil rig six miles off the California coast near Santa Barbara sprang a leak and in a mere 12 hours spread copious amounts of oil over a 100 square mile area. Interestingly, the many primitive methods (such as soaps, boons, rollers, burning) used in attempting to control the problem have all failed. Man was ready to drill for oil on the continental shelf, but he was not ready to cope with the problems brought forth by a leak in the system.

How much oil, DDT, and other pollutants will it take to foul the environment of vital microscopic plant life? No one knows, but until man does know can he continue to pollute at an ever increasing rate? The question is still awaiting an answer.

Water Pollution and Health Hazards

Insofar as threats to public health are concerned, there is little factual evidence of ill effects resulting directly from pollution of communities' water supplies aside from those that stem from the presence of pathogenic and parasitic organisms. However, research centering on nitrates from fertilizers (previously mentioned as water pollutants from agriculture) has shown that infiltrating the human tissue they become nitrites which rob the blood of oxygen. Like carbon dioxide these nitrites are known to tie up hemoglobin in the blood, replacing oxygen and so becoming a cause of methemoglobinemia, which results in infant cyanosis.

Some of the indirect effects of water pollution on health, such as the potential oxygen cycle disruption, are also under study. Currently a group of United States ecologists are conducting a series of studies with Eskimos. Apparently, oil spills originating on Alaska's north shore have resulted in oil being trapped in the narrow space between the water and ice, killing the plankton. This could present a very serious problem in the Eskimo's food chain cycle, since the bears and seals who provide the major food supply for the Eskimo feed directly on the fish and mollusks, whose food supply is the plankton. If the plankton are destroyed the whole food chain would be disrupted, which could have disastrous effects on the final member of that chain—the Eskimo.

It appears that man can no longer take such cycles for granted. No longer can he afford to take for granted the quality of the water in the sea, nor, for that matter, the quality and quantity of the water that flows from his kitchen tap.

Suggestions for Individual Action

- Support legislation and bond issues that provide for proper sewage disposal and the elimination of cesspools and septic tanks in the community.
- Insure that only limited application of salt be permitted on streets to prevent icing. This salt can cause damage to lawns, trees and water resources.
- Develop an ecological conscience based on a concern for the quality of the environment. This must include a redefinition of "progress" toward an emphasis on long term quality rather than immediate quantity.

1. Develop a paper describing the method of sewage disposal being used in your community. Consider such factors as the system's adequacy, or plans to improve the system and resultant costs.
2. Develop a paper focusing on the interrelationship of population and pollution problems.
3. Develop a listing of all possible sources of water pollution in your community. Include such pertinent facts as type of pollution and location of the sources.
4. Read a book (refer to bibliography) or article in a professional journal dealing with the air pollution problem and give your reaction to the material you have read.
5. What measures has the federal government taken to insure the quality and availability of water in the nation?

CHAPTER 6

Noise Pollution, Radiation
and Pesticides

Noise Pollution

Noise means unwanted sounds. It has its origin in two Latin words: nausea, which means sick, and noxia, which means harm. In New York City persons first show evidence of hearing loss at age 25. In Africa the age is 70. Human hearing begins to be damaged by prolonged exposure to more than 85 decibels of noise on the A scale. Noise from heavy city traffic has been found to measure at 90 decibels. The sources of noise pollution are many. Traffic, construction, sirens, fans, air conditioners, radios, and crowds of people—all make their impact in a modern world of noise, and present man with a very special problem. In most cases he has no way of turning it off or immediately escaping from it. But noise can be controlled. Acoustical engineers have the technology to accomplish this. Most machines can be acoustically designed in such a manner that the sounds they produce can be greatly diminished.

A Special Problem—The SST's. The development of the new SST's (supersonic transports) presents a possible world health crisis in a number of ways. The problem of the sonic boom that people in a 50-60 mile path below the plane may hear is receiving much attention. Secretary Alan Boyd has said, "In simple terms the fight over the SST raises old questions of controlling the effect of technology on the environment. I am convinced we have long since passed the point where we can make transportation decisions affecting any or all forms of transportation without weighing in advance their social as well as their economic impact upon communities and the regions they serve."[8]

Noise pollution is a health problem. It is also a solvable problem. Man need only to apply what he knows to quiet the problem.

Effects of Loud Noise. Loud noises are known to affect the body in a number of ways, depending on the situation and the severity of the noise. Some of the known effects are:

---

8. "News and Comments, The SST and The Government: Critics Shout into a Vacuum," *Science*, September 8, 1967, p. 1147.

- Paling of the skin
- Constriction of blood vessels
- Tensing of muscles
- Secretion of adrenal hormones
- Nervous tension
- Increased blood pressure

Radiation, Man and His Environment

From the beginning of time man has been exposed to forms of natural radiation, the most common being cosmic radiation from the sun. This source of radiation has presented man with health problems relative to skin cancer and certain other suspected disorders. The American Medical Association has voiced concern over the potential dangers to human health from overexposure to the sun's rays, especially such as result from prolonged or excessive sunbathing.

The Nature of Radiation. Radiation is a form of energy transport, while the process of radioactivity describes the nuclei of certain specific elements undergoing spontaneous disintegration or decay and as a consequence liberating energy in the form of alpha, beta or gamma particles.

Radiation, released into the environment, can penetrate tissue and produce chemical changes in the cells. The degree of damage depends on the source of radioactivity and the length of exposure.

Rapidly developing cells of the body are particularly susceptible to the destructive action radiation and radioactivity generate. Genetic material, which governs most of the cellular processes, including its reproductive function, is especially sensitive to radiation exposure. This is particularly true in the germinal cells of human and animal testes and ova.

Man Harnesses This Form of Energy. The medical use of radiation in the form of diagnosis and treatment of certain disorders also has its potential dangers. In terms of the principle that all unnecessary radiation must be avoided, X-ray exposures should be made only when a physician or dentist deems them necessary for proper diagnosis or treatment. Recent efforts have been made to hold the amount of exposure necessary for such usage to a minimal level commensurate with the amount considered functional for the purposes intended.

Radium dial pocket watches, a source of radiation emission, have met with restrictive sales legislation in New York City, since such watches are usually worn near the waistline, thus exposing the reproductive organs to possible danger. It should also be noted that radium-painted dials on clocks are a potential hazard if the radioactive element found on the dial is ingested. Such materials should be kept away from children who might inhale or eat flakes of paint from the dial of a discarded or broken clock.

Television picture tubes, especially those on color sets, give off soft radiation very much like that produced by X-ray machines, with a lower penetrating power, however. Shields have been built into the set to protect the viewer from being exposed to these rays. Recently, radiation leaks have been found to exist in some of the color sets due to inadequate shielding and corrective measures have been established.

Radiation from the Peaceful Use of Atomic Energy. With the total energy requirements in the U. S. increasing at a rate of about 3 1/4 percent a year and the demands on electricity nearly doubling every ten years, man has increasingly turned to the atom to meet the need for greater energy sources.

Most evident has been the use of atomic energy for the generating of electricity. Presently the electric generating capacity of the United States is 250-260 million kilowatts. By 1980 this figure will have reached a projected 520 million kilowatts and by the year 2000 the anticipated figure is 1.6 billion kilowatts.

Nuclear power plants have been built and are operating in various parts of the United States. Some have encountered stiff resistance from local conservation and other naturalist groups. The major problem results from the fact that some radioactive contamination of water occurs as a result of seepage through small imperfections in the metal tubes containing the uranium fuel. Periodically, these wastes are drawn off, treated and buried.

Peaceful Use of Nuclear Explosions. Nuclear explosions have been used in facilitating the availability of natural gas supplies, as in Project Gasbuggy (1967) in New Mexico, an offshoot of the Atomic Energy Commission's program "to develop peaceful uses for nuclear explosives," known as operation "Plowshare." The project has come up with ideas for using nuclear explosives to build dams, harbors, canals and stimulate both natural gas and oil production. (In relation to Project Gasbuggy, however, the Public Health Service found that the radioactivity of vegetation downwind from the blast was increased ten times.)

The contamination problems involved in such projects are obviously very complex, and it remains a simple fact that even though nuclear explosions may be a more efficent and effective way to get the job done, no matter how peaceful the objective, they nevertheless produce radioactivity. One must question the worth of efficiency achieved in this way as opposed to the possible consequences it has relative to the quality of the environment.

Fallout from Nuclear Explosions. Fallout refers to radioactive debris that settles to the surface of the earth following nuclear explosions. Since most organisms living on earth are now vulnerable for exposure to detectable radiation resulting from a single nuclear explosion, there has been great interest and utmost concern as to the possible effects of fallout on living organisms, including the human population.

How much of a contributor fallout from nuclear explosions (test or otherwise) is to world air pollution problems hinges on many factors. The characteristics of fallout resulting from specific explosions are determined by two factors: (1) the height of the burst and (2) the size or power of the explosion. These factors determine whether the fallout takes on the characteristics of early (local) fallout which occurs in the first twenty-four hours following an explosion, or worldwide (delayed) fallout.

Bursts which occur at great heights and do not suck up dust or water into the fireball produce little or no local fallout. Instead the contaminated particles condense in very small, very soluble particles. These are widely dispersed and descend to earth, ultimately as part of what is called worldwide fallout, which is characterized as either "tropospheric" or "stratospheric" fallout.

Detonation of low yield devices (less than a few hundred kilotons) at or near the surface of the earth project their fission products no higher than the troposphere. Tropospheric fallout is washed down by rain or snow within one day to four weeks. Since winds travel mainly in a west-east direction (in the Northern Hemisphere), tropospheric fallout reaches the earth in an irregular band roughly centered at about the same latitude as the detonation.

High yield explosions propel their fission products into the stratosphere. There is no agreement as to exactly how, when, and where these radioactive particles descend from the stratosphere to the troposphere, then to the earth. Months or years later it descends into the troposphere near the gap in the tropopause. This sinking is accelerated in late winter and spring.

It should be noted however that recent studies have shown a tendency for the stratospheric fallout to descend earthward in a matter of months, depending on the geographic location and the time of explosion. A considerable amount of hazardous radioactivity remains in fallout when it reaches the earth.[9]

In early testing important mistakes were made in judging the medical hazards of such fallout and the risk of genetic damage was dismissed. However by 1957, a report of the Atomic Energy Commission Biological and Medical Advisory Committee had concluded that fallout from tests completed to date would probably result in 2,300 to 13,000 cases of serious genetic defects per year throughout the world population.[10]

---

9. Barry Commoner, *Science and Survival* (New York: Viking Press, 1967), p. 17.
10. Ibid., p. 18.

Pesticides and Pollution

Rachel Carson in her widely read book "Silent Spring" called man's attention in no uncertain terms to the great dangers inherent in the use of pesticides. There is abundant evidence proving that both man and wildlife encounter ill effects resulting from the use of certain pesticides. In some instances the soil has become polluted with these toxicants for many years. Fish in Lake Michigan were, for example, found to contain the deadly poison DDT. The Michigan Department of Agriculture in the summer of 1969 found some of the fish to be so poisoned with DDT that they found it necessary to confiscate tons of Coho salmon considered unfit for human consumption. In recognition of facts like these, certain pesticides such as DDT have already met with legislative restrictions in various parts of the United States.

There is little question that pesticides have contributed to the nation's food productivity, but at the same time they pose a threat to both man and his wildlife. One of the major problems centers on pesticides entering the cyclic processes of natural food chains. Consider the following: A farmer sprays a weak level of DDT on his crops to kill damaging bugs. The bugs ingest the DDT along with the plant matter and die. DDT is a "hard" pesticide which means it will not break down quickly into harmless substances; rather, it will persist and build up in the organism. If an insect-eating bird devours the pesticide-laden bugs, the pesticide will enter the tissues of its body. If the bird eats quantities of the bugs, as most birds do in a short period of time, the pesticide will accumulate in the tissues, and since pesticides such as DDT are not excreted by the body, this accumulation will continue and gain in concentration.

The concentration is thus magnified in the tissues of the bird. It may or may not kill the bird, but, in any event, continues to build in concentration as it moves along the food chain.

In some cases, the pesticides do not directly kill a predator in a long food chain, but rather interferes with certain vital processes. Bald eagles have fallen victims to pesticides several ways. Of a large number of bald eagles found dead or incapacitated over a 3 year period, almost all showed high levels of DDT in their tissues. In other cases DDT accumulation seemed to interfere with the female eagle's ability to make a good strong shell for her eggs. In some instances the shells could not take the natural pressures of incubation which resulted in cracked shells and death to the embryos.

Man's exposure to pesticides may, on the other hand, occur in a variety of ways other than through ingestion from the food chain. Farm workers, as a notable example, involved in the direct application of pesticides, have been a victim of some of the most damaging exposures.

While studies have indicated the potential dangers of pesticides upon various organisms, the problem remains a complex one. Of utmost concern is the somewhat frightening fact that the more subtle, indirect and long range effects of these pesticides and herbicides upon both man and wildlife are not known. The effects of the ingestion of small amounts of these chemical pollutants are also not fully understood.

Pesticides and Water Pollution. Pesticides also endanger man through his water supply. These pollutants may enter the water supply by way of:

1. Direct application to the water surface.
2. Drifting onto the water surface from adjoining treated areas.
3. Being washed in from the watershed.

With the amount of such chemicals being used, it seems inevitable that some of the materials should ultimately find their way to waterways and even penetrate into the underground aquifers. A number of startling examples already are a record, such as the following:

Montebello, California: In June 1945, a small plant in Alhambra, California began manufacturing 2,4-D: A batch of the raw material failed to react properly and the chemicals were dumped inadvertently into a sewer. Thence, this waste entered the Alhambra pumping station, passed through the Tri-Cities activated sludge sewage treatment plant, and was discharged into a mile-long ditch. From here the contaminant traveled some 3 to 5 miles above ground, then seeped into the underground strata from which Montebello, a city of about 25,000 population, obtained its water supply. Within 17 days after the manufacture of the weed killer started, taste and odor of a chemical used in the manufacture, 2,4-D dichlorophenol, was noticed in the eleven wells supplying the City. The operation of the plant was stopped within 30 days, yet the taste and odor of dichlorophenol persisted for 4 to 5 years. This case is interesting and important because it shows the possible long-time effects from wastes even though they were unwisely discharged over a relatively short period.[11]

South Platte River Basin Near Henderson, Colo.: This represents another significant and historic case in the serious pollution of underground water. As a war measure in 1943, the Rocky Mt. Arsenal of the Chemical Corps, located immediately north of Stapleton Municipal Airport, Denver, started to manufacture warfare agents. In 1955, the arsenal was leased to the Shell Oil Company which has used the plant to manufacture insecticides. Five different oil refineries and two manufacturing concerns have operated in close proximity.

It seems probable that sludge from the pond used at the arsenal by the chemical Corps between 1943 and 1955, to hold chemical waste effluents, is the source of the contamination. Phytotoxic substances in this waste included chlorates and phosphonates. It appears that other waste substances in the discharge in the presence of air, water and sunlight caused these waste

---

11. U. S. Department of Health, Education, and Welfare, Proceedings: The National Conference on Water Pollution, Washington, D. C., 1960, pp. 230-31.

materials to combine and form 2,4-D. There is no evidence to indicate that the herbicide 2,4-D had been purposefully manufactured at the arsenal. We must assume, therefore, that the 2,4-D was synthesized in the waste mixture from precursors introduced from the plant operation. There may also be other contaminants.

The first farm crops to be affected were in 1951. It apparently took 7 to 8 years for the contaminated water to travel approximately 3 miles. By 1958, contaminated water extended in an area of several square miles and seriously affected crop production, industry, and the people who had relied on the water for their own culinary purposes and for livestock. At least one case of illness has been shown to have been caused by drinking this polluted water. The area within this acquifer basin, much of which is not yet affected, is said to cover some 60 square miles. How long this pollution of poisons will last and what total damage yet will result is unknown, but obviously it will be many years before the damage is corrected. Many shallow and some deep wells occur within this basin, and approximately 150 residences are within the known or suspected area of contaminated shallow ground water. No information now is available on the course and rate of flow of the contaminated water arriving in the vicinity of South Platte River.[12]

The Proceedings of the National Center on Water Pollution of the U. S. Department of Health, Education, and Welfare drew the following conclusions relative to the problem of pesticides:

The enormous and ever growing quantity and kinds of extremely toxic, broad spectrum, stable chemicals used as pesticides throughout America give warning that an objective forward look is necessary. If our people are to receive protection as well as benefit from the mature and safe use of these needed pesticides, there must be more advanced planning and better coordination in the management and use of chemical controls. I believe that dangerous and costly pollution of both surface and ground water with these poisons is inevitable unless effective steps are promptly taken. Recent case histories of pollution confirm this view and show that such contamination may be serious and its correction slow and costly. Because of the nature of the problem, more effective controls must be placed on the distribution and use of dangerous toxicants at the source. This, I believe, should include more effective testing, registration, labeling, and distribution of poisons. I am convinced that we need a clearer declaration of national policy by Congress and by many States regulating the use of pesticides in the broad public interest. More effective coordination must be obtained between agencies and interests directing control and those groups and agencies of State and Federal Government, as well as national and local interests, that are vitally affected by operational programs.

There is critical need for more adequate support of basic research. Many costly mistakes and controversies of the past have been kindled through

---

12.   Ibid., p. 231.

a painful lack of facts on which to act. Sound research should precede an operational program of control and eradication.

It is apparent that the establishment of safe limits of toxicants in water is an involved and long-term undertaking. Yet safe and clearly defined standards for water quality are needed. It is essential that public and private forces unite to support a coordinated program of research.

A few additional "needs" are submitted for consideration—

1. To the extent possible, use toxicants that are selective that will give reasonable control of a particular pest and do the least damage to desirable forms of life.
2. Give more emphasis to biological and cultural controls.
3. When chemical controls are necessary, use formulations, methods of application (i.e., mode of treatment and carrier), time of treatment, and dosage that will be the least damaging to the biota.
4. Use toxicants that hydrolize promptly and those that can be utilizied or broken down by organisms in the soil.
5. Use spot and not broadcast treatment wherever possible.
6. Determine toxicity of runoff and seepage water for different materials, dosages, and modes of pesticide application.
7. Determine the toxicity of the toxicant to the various organisms in the environment.
8. Direct research toward side or indirect effects of various pesticides.
9. Develop more specific controls.
10. Study the total environment and its managements so that control can be carried on more wisely.

Pesticides and Human Health. It must be pointed out that there are many conflicting reports regarding the hazards of certain pesticides to human health. There is evidence however that indicates man's tissues to be so contaminated by pesticides (especially DDT) that his body would have to be considered "unfit" as a source of food.

There is also evidence that DDT is being found in the breast milk of humans. DDT levels in human milk in the United States have been found to range from .15 to .25 parts per million.[13] The maximum daily intake of DDT recommended by the United Nations is four times *less* than this figure. This level of DDT in human milk is also five times the amount allowed in the interstate shipment of cows' milk.

It is very clear that man must restrict the use of certain pesticides until further research yields more exacting information as to its potential hazards to human health. To continue the use of these pesticides without full knowledge of their possible ill effects on man and the environment is a folly we can no longer afford.

---

13. Frank Graham, Jr., *Since Silent Spring*, Boston, Houghton Mifflin Co., 1970, p. 149.

Suggestions for Individual Action

- Do not purchase or use long-lived pesticides such as those containing chlorinated hydrocarbons (DDT, etc.).
- Consider using "natural" alternatives in pest control before using chemical poisons.
- If you must use a chemical poison, follow these guidelines: Use only recommended dosages and only at the proper time of year. Never apply chemicals near food or water sources.
- Remove weeds by hand rather than by applying herbicides.

1. What are some of the major sources of noise pollution in your local community? What can be done to lessen the problem?
2. What measures has the federal government taken to protect the general public from possible radiation hazards?
3. What measures have been taken by the federal government and your local state government (if any) to restrict the use of pesticides?
4. How much radiation can the human body normally tolerate without fear of the hazards of exposure? How is this determined?

CHAPTER 7

The Environment
and the Quality of Life

The creation of an environment in which scientific technology renders man completely independent of natural forces calls to mind a dismal future in which man will be served by robots and therefore himself becomes a robot.

The humanness of life depends above all on the quality of man's relationships to the rest of creation—to the winds and stars, to the flowers and beasts, to smiling and weeping humanity.

—RENÉ DUBOS

Attempting to set criteria for a high quality environment is a monumental task. Since the beginning of recorded time man has searched for his Utopia. While modern man has interpreted Utopia to mean a "perfect state," it is interesting to note that it has its origin in the Greek word meaning "nowhere."

There are however some factors that appear to be essential to the quality of any human environment. The factors of environmental health, environmental space and environmental diversity all seem to fall into this category. The quality of "humanness" found in man also seems to be an essential factor.

In working toward a quality environment man must consider a broad spectrum of factors. Rats in the ghetto, a hungry child, overcrowding and improper sanitation are all environmental problems.

Consider the problem of rats in ghetto areas. Extermination procedures such as the placing of poisons and the setting of traps do not solve the problem. They are simply measures aimed at reducing or controlling the size of the rat population. The most effective way of ridding an area of rats is to eliminate their nesting sites and their source of food. Is this possible in a ghetto area without making extensive changes in the total environment?

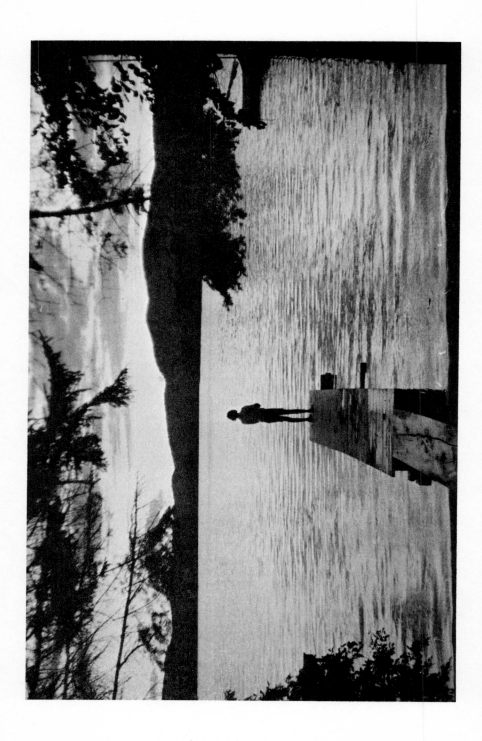

A Point of Reference—Toward a Solution. The environmental problems facing modern man are in the form of dilemmas and risks stemming from the overwhelming advances in science and technology at a time when man seems to lack adequate tools of insight and wisdom for dealing with all aspects of them wisely. For the major portion of his existence on earth man has been a food gatherer living off the fruits of his environment, rather than dominating it.

But man is beginning to take note of those natural forces that must remain intact in order for him to survive—that he can no longer change or remove at will. Perhaps most important is the realization that life processes involve the expenditure of energy and thus the relationship between an organism and its environment must be considered a problem of energy exchange—a *balanced* energy exchange. For example, the human food supply is the function of an amount of energy received from the sun by the plant cover on earth, and the efficiency with which that energy is converted to carbohydrates usable by man. What is essential then is a new understanding of the relationship between biology and society; to reach a new set of checks and balances between man, his sciences and the environment in which he lives.

Thus we enter on the whole issue at stake, be it local or worldwide, air pollution or other environmental problems, whether man can carry out his life processes and all that goes with them and still maintain a biological balance that will keep the planet Earth in habitable condition.

The Future—Some Bright Spots

To keep the earth's atmosphere suitable for maintaining life, and the earth itself in a habitable condition, requires international cooperation. Fortunately this cooperation is beginning to become reality in many ways.

A United Nations Conference on Human Environment for 1972 has been approved by the U. N. General Assembly. The draft resolution entitled "The Problems of Human Environment" proposed this special international forum. According to the Swedish ambassador, Sverker Astrom: "If only a fraction of those resources in the form of brain-power, technical know-how, equipment and capital which are now devoted to the perfection of the means of mass destruction were released to be utilized for social purposes, for the rational planning of the human environment in urban and rural areas, then the total gain in terms of human happiness and of social justice would be enormous. . . ."

Such a conference is indeed a step in the right direction, especially if it can generate action and cooperation on a worldwide scale. It is also worth noting that an exchange of United States and U.S.S.R. delegations for air and water pollution is a new addition to the Scientific, Technical, Educational and Cultural Exchange program between the two nations.

National Legislation. Legislation regarding environmental conditions and restrictions in the United States needs to be expanded further, on a broad national scale. Owing to the very nature of air and water pollution it would be ineffectual and utterly futile for each state to establish its own policy. This would lead (at the very least) to industries locating in states where less restrictive control measures existed, or to conflict between adjoining states over the pollution of a common river, or the drifting of a contaminated air mass over state lines.

Dr. Sidney Galler of the Smithsonian Institute centered in on the role of the federal government relative to environmental problems as he testified before the Senate Interior Committee. He stated:

Throughout the history of the world, various nations have risen and fallen in accordance with overexploitation and deterioration of their resource bases. If we are to avoid the same pitfall, we must provide a scientific foundation for conservation, development and effective use of our resources. It is essential to our survival as a Nation to take effective action on these problems.

We need a broad new program of Federally supported ecological research. With our resources gradually disappearing and with our capacity to destroy the environment growing each day, we must know the impact on our environment of every step we take from now on.

We must know in advance that wiping out forests destroys the soil, ruins lakes and streams, even affects the climate and causes some agricultural crops to die. We must know that digging a canal to the ocean can admit sea lampreys and wipe out our lake trout fishery. We must know that phosphates in detergents will fill our likes with fast growing algae.

If we are to do these things—if we are to save the natural resources of this land to sustain ourselves and future generations—then we must begin at once to develop the governmental programs and institutions which will accomplish that life or death goal.[14]

Federal legislation regarding air pollution took a giant step forward with the passage of The Clean Air Act of 1963. It authorized the federal government to establish national standards for the control of emissions from gasoline-powered vehicles. It has also given the government authority to take action in cases of interstate pollution.

Still unresolved are such questions as how to deal with contaminated air masses moving over state boundaries. Also unresolved are questions of uniform air quality and emission standards. These still are in the process of determination and development.

The President's Committee on Population

On July 16, 1968 former President Lyndon B. Johnson issued the following mandate to the Committee on Population and Family Planning:

---

14. Proceedings: The National Conference on Air Pollution, Washington, D. C., 1966. p. 453.

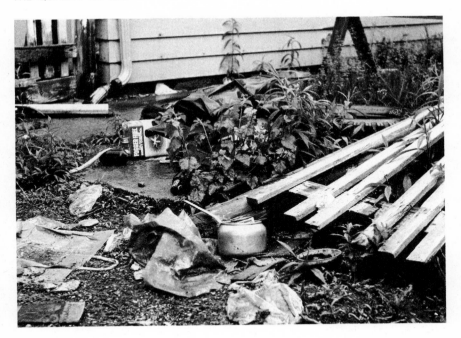

Man leaves his mark on the environment. Such sights have become too
common as man continues to ignore the condition of his environment.

I am appointing a Committee of distinguished citizens and Government
officials to make a careful review of Federal policies and programs in relation to worldwide and domestic needs.

I am asking the Committee
— to determine ways of providing the American people with meaningful
   information about population change and assuring that its significance
   will be understood by the rising generation.
— to define the Federal Government's direct role in research and training
   in population matters including the physiology of human reproduction,
   in fertility control and the development of new contraceptives, and
   the Government's role in supporting such research and training in
   private institutions at home and overseas.
— to define the responsibility of the Federal Government, in cooperation with State, community, and private agencies in assuring that all
   families have access to information and services that will enable them
   to plan the number and spacing of their children.
— to suggest actions which the United States should take in concert with
   other countries and with international organizations to help the developing countries of the world to understand and to deal effectively
   with their high rates of population growth.
I am asking the Committee to provide me with an estimate of the costs
of an effective five-year program plan in research, training and services.

The Committee may establish working groups of government and non-government experts to study technical, economic or social aspects of the population problem.

I am asking the Committee to report to me within 120 days.
THE WHITE HOUSE
July 16, 1968

The Committee, once formed, acted promptly to submit its first set of recommendations. The following are quoted from the recommendations made by the President's Committee on Population and Family Planning:

November, 1968
POPULATION AND FAMILY PLANNING:
THE TRANSITION FROM
CONCERN TO ACTION
PROPOSALS
FOR IMMEDIATE CONSIDERATION

The world's population problems must be high on the world's agenda. In the more developed nations, present rates of population growth cannot continue indefinitely without causing serious social and environmental problems. The rapid growth rates of the developing nations are a threat to their own plans for economic and social progress, on which the peace of the world may well depend. In both, the level of information and understanding must be improved. In both, the very quality of life is at stake.

No simple program will resolve the world's population problems: They demand a variety of actions on a sustained basis by governments, private organizations, and individuals. This report recommends a broad range of actions by the Government of the United States to resolve pressing problems and to establish sound, long-range policies. Present problems are so urgent, however, that the Committee has selected from the full report the following key proposals, recommended for immediate consideration.

❖   ❖   ❖   ❖

As its first responsibility, the Committee considered domestic programs in population and family planning intended primarily to further the health and welfare of the American people. The Committee is convinced, moreover, that sound domestic programs will increase our experience and knowledge, and in consequence will make our participation in international programs more useful and valued. The Committee, therefore, recommends:

1. That the Federal Government expand family planning programs to make information and services available by 1973 on a voluntary basis to all American women who want but cannot afford them.

This policy will require an increase in the Federal appropriation for domestic family planning services, to be provided on a strictly voluntary basis, from $30 million in the fiscal year 1969 to $150 million in 1973. This is a small price to pay for providing help to an estimated five million women now deprived by poverty and ignorance of the opportunity to plan their families effectively.

2. That the Department of Health, Education, and Welfare and the Office of Economic Opportunity develop specific five-year plans for their population and family planning programs.

The task to be done is so complex that a detailed, long-range plan is essential for translating policy into day-to-day operations. A prospectus for such a plan is presented in the full report.

3. That the Office of Education provide significant assistance to appropriate education agencies in the development of materials on population and family life.

All levels of the educational system stand in need of materials and curricula on the causes and consequences of population change, so that the American people can confront population issues intelligently. Also needed are curricula on family life so that personal decisions about marriage and parenthood can be made responsibly and with adequate information. Federal assistance for local education programs in these fields should be expanded rapidly to at least $8 million annually.

*   *   *   *

Beyond this nation's domestic needs, the United States shares with other nations a concern about the world's population problems. Increasing numbers of countries, caught in the crisis of rapid population growth, recognize that their aspirations for a better life may be frustrated without effective population and family planning programs. Assisting such programs is now an integral part of our national commitment to help the developing countries. The Committe therefore recommends:

4. That the United States continue to expand its programs of international assistance in population and family planning as rapidly as funds can be properly allocated by the U.S. and effectively utilized by recipient countries and agencies.

Reducing population growth is not a substitute for economic development. And yet in most of the developing countries, a decline in birth rates is necessary if they are to satisfy the reasonable aspirations of their people. Programs in population should continue to have high priority and increasing support as part of general assistance to social and economic development. It is clear now that our expenditures for assistance in this field should grow substantially in the next three to five years; however, the amount and allocation of increase should depend on a continuing review of our efforts in this field and the scale and effectiveness of programs undertaken by the developing countries.

5. That experienced specialists from other countries be invited to serve on advisory groups for both our domestic and international programs.

The American contribution to population programs abroad can only be a small part of their total costs, so it must be allocated through a carefully considered set of priorities to maximize long-term effects. This allocation will be more effective if the Federal Government seeks the advice of experts from other countries, some of which have more experience with large-scale family planning programs than our own country. Americans have served on such advisory groups for other countries; we should seek in return the benefit of similar advice for both our domestic and international programs.

*   *   *   *

Additional research and a greater supply of trained personnel are essential for both domestic and foreign programs. Larger research programs, especially when combined with the recommended expansion of service programs, will create a demand for qualified personnel and for programs to train them. The Committee therefore recommends:

6. That the newly established Center for Population Research accelerate the Federal Government's research and training programs in both the biological and social sciences and that within two years the Center be expanded into a National Institute for Population Research, established by act of Congress.
The expanded program of biomedical and social science research and training in population supported by the National Institute of Child Health and Human Development and coordinated by its Center for Population Research should rise to $30 million in the fiscal year 1970 and to $100 million in 1971. This level of funding will enable the Center to launch much needed programs on improved methods of contraception, basic research on the physiology of reproduction and social science research integral to population problems. The Center should become the focal point within the government for information about population research and training, whether domestic or foreign. Planning should begin now to bring about its transformation into a separate National Institute for Population Research within the next two years.
7. That the Federal Government provide basic support for population studies centers.
Priority should be given to basic support for existing population centers primarily in universities to carry out research and training programs in the biomedical, health and social sciences. Support should also be given to the establishment of additional university centers. Such support will attract scientists, teachers and administrators by assuring them of career opportunities. Basic support for existing and additional centers, including construction, is estimated at an average annual cost of $40 million.

❖   ❖   ❖   ❖

Making family planning available and effective is a principal aim of the actions recommended for immediate consideration, but family planning is only one of the important influences on population change. Population trends are influenced profoundly by many other things—for example, by tax policies, participation of women in the labor force, job and housing opportunities, population mobility, and marriage rates. Unfortunately, both knowledge and public information about population trends and policies are limited. The present report, completed in four months, should be supplemented by a more thorough review. The Committee therefore recommends:
8. That Congress authorize and the President appoint a Commission on Population.
Such a Commission should make the American public aware of the economic, educational and social impact of population trends. It should analyze the consequences of alternative U.S. policies in the light of this country's determination to enhance the quality of American life. It should evaluate the progress of this nation's programs and review the extent to which the recommendations of this Committee have been implemented. The Commission could have a major impact in highlighting for the American people the urgency and importance of the population problem.

These proposals have received significant attention and some have been put into action. Only July 18, 1969 President Richard Nixon in a message to the first session of the Ninety-first Congress called for the establishment of a Commission on Population Growth and the American Future. In doing so he stated:

The Congress should give the Commission responsibility for inquiry and recommendations in three specific areas.

First, *the probable course of population growth, internal migration and related demographic developments between now and the year 2000.*

As much as possible, these projections should be made by regions, states, and metropolitan areas. Because there is an element of uncertainty in such projections, various alternative possibilities should be plotted.

It is of special importance to note that, beginning in August of 1970, population data by county will become available from the decennial census, which will have been taken in April of that year. By April 1971, computer summaries of first-count data will be available by census tract and an important range of information on income, occupations, education, household composition, and other vital consideration will also be in hand. The Federal government can make better use of such demographic information than it has done in the past, and state governments and other political subdivisions can also use such data to better advantage. The Commission on Population Growth and the American Future will be an appropriate instrument for this important initiative.

Second, *the resources in the public sector of the economy that will be required to deal with the anticipated growth in population.*

The single greatest failure of foresight—at all levels of government—over the past generation has been in areas connected with expanding population. Government and legislatures have frequently failed to appreciate the demands which continued population growth would impose on the public sector. These demands are myriad: they will range from pre-school classrooms to post-doctoral fellowships; from public works which carry water over thousands of miles to highways which carry people and products from region to region; from vest pocket parks in crowded cities to forest preserves and quiet lakes in the countryside. Perhaps especially, such demands will assert themselves in forms that affect the quality of life. The time is at hand for a serious assessment of such needs.

Third, *ways in which population growth may affect the activities of Federal, state and local governments.*

In some respects, population growth affects everything that American government does. Yet only occasionally do our governmental units pay sufficient attention to population growth in their own planning. Only occasionally do they consider the serious implications of demographic trends for their present and future activities.

Yet some of the necessary information is at hand and can be made available to all levels of government. Much of the rest will be obtained by the Commission. For such information to be of greatest use, however, it should also be interpreted and analyzed and its implications should be made more evident. It is particularly in this connection that the work of the Commission on Population Growth and the American Future will be as much educational as investigative. The American public and its governing units are not as alert as they should be to these growing challenges. A responsible but insistent voice of reason and foresight is needed. The Commission can provide that voice in the years immediately before us.

The membership of the Commission should include two members from each house of the Congress, together with knowledgeable men and women who are broadly representative of our society. The majority should be citizens who have demonstrated a capacity to deal with important questions of public policy. The membership should also include specialists in the biological, social, and environmental sciences, in theology and law, in the arts and in engineering. The Commission should be empowered to create advisory panels to consider subdivisions of its broad subject area and to invite experts and leaders from all parts of the world to join these panels in their deliberations.

The Commission should be provided with an adequate staff and budget, under the supervision of an executive director of exceptional experience and understanding.

In order that the Commission will have time to utilize the initial data which results from the 1970 census, I ask that it be established for a period of two years. An interim report to the President and Congress should be required at the end of the first year.

Education—A Solution to the Population Crisis

The most humane solution to the population problem seems to have its foundation in the educational processes of the nation. To recognize the population crisis as a problem of high priority for the survival of mankind is to acknowledge that it is at least partially the responsibility of education and educators to bring it within the bounds of control.

The United States public has been vague, naive and relatively ignorant of the population problem.[15] Even some of those deeply concerned with the problems of air and water pollution, shortage of natural resources, and so on, have failed to recognize that over-population is the major problem—the others resulting directly from this primary problem. Dr. Robert Rienon, Professor of Political Science at the State University of New York at Albany, recently made the following statement: "The abuses to the environment are the consequences of a set of forces foremost of which is that of population. Changing values so that the population can be limited, by fiat if necessary, is the only hope for our species."[16]

It is quite clear in the literature that those concerned with a humane solution to the problem of population see the possibility for solution in a public educated to fully comprehend the population crisis, and to recognize its own responsibilities towards making the attempt to alleviate that problem. If education has a responsibility to shape, or at least to influence the society in which it exists . . . it has never had a more critical task than the one that awaits it in the matter of population control. If education is to tackle the problem of teaching directed toward "reproductive responsibility," it must concern itself directly with the attitudes and values of the individual in society. It must strive to help the individual make a change in attitude and behavior in relation to

15. "The American Public Looks at the Population Crisis," Population Reference Bureau, Inc., 16 February 1966, p. 2.
16. T. H. Littlefield, "A Gloomy Future Seen by Environment Experts," Albany *Times-Union*, 28 September 1969, p. 4B.

the population problem. A change that may be possible if the educational process were to aim its programs at helping each individual to know and understand the following:

- The major cause of population growth in the United States is the rapid decrease in the death rate, without a corresponding decrease in the birth rate. A population growth rate of "0" must be the ultimate goal of population control.
- The nature of the population problem and its relationship to problems of pollution, mental health, transportation and medical services.
- It is clearly necessary to solve the population problem in a humane way or nature will solve it her way, be it through war, pestilence, disease or mass starvation.
- The value of humanness is the prime value, and it is in relation to human worth and human value that the decisions about population must be made.

A Redefinition of Progress—To Save the Environment

Some see the solution to the environmental problem in changing the human value structure. Dr. Rienon has urged that we redefine progress. "To redefine progress demands I believe an exchange of values. I think we must exchange, not an affluent life for a poor one, but rather pure air for less goods; a swimming hole instead of a swimming pool. . . ."[17]

To suggest a changing of human values and a redefinition of progress may seem like asking for the impossible. But the very nature of the problems of population and pollution have their origin in the human value system and the powerful drive of modern progress. What is needed in relation to the environment is a rebirth of a sense of community spirit . . . a rebirth that can only occur deep in the mind of man.

Dr. René Dubos, speaking to foreign diplomats and State Department officials, warned that "Pollution is not self-regulating. If we leave it alone, we face disaster in part or in general. Change will come only from fear of worse disasters than those that might occur.[18] The fear is beginning to become evident and action is starting to take place. But it seems insane that man should wait until he has put the entire planet in jeopardy before he starts to act. The delayed action on the part of man may well prove to be the final fatal blow to the species if delayed any longer.

---

17. Ibid.
18. "U. S. Plans Internation Environmental Conference," *Environmental Science and Technology,* January 1969, p. 9.

A Call to Action: A View Toward Change

It is simply not enough to be aware and concerned about the environmental crisis. The need is for action—action by you, for it is within the means of each individual to do something about it. Society at large has been charged with the crime of gross neglect of the environment. But who is society? Is it not a conglomerate of individual human beings? Municipalities, industries and governmental agencies have also been charged with the crime of gross neglect of the environment. Can such innate organizations be held responsible or should the responsibility fall directly on the shoulders of the many individuals that together make up these organizations?

It is clear to this writer that in order for there to be any meaningful changes relative to population growth and pollution control in the United States the attitudes, values and actions of individual human beings must first be altered. The changes necessary in our society to save its environmental health will come of themselves when each *individual* acts as an intelligent, selfless and responsible human being. There cannot be an "ecologically sound" society until there are many such persons.

A SELECTED BIBLIOGRAPHY

POPULATION

DAY, LINCOLN H. *Too Many Americans*. Boston: Houghton Mifflin Company, 1964.

EHRLICH, PAUL R. *The Population Bomb*. New York: Ballantine Books, Inc., 1965.

HARDIN, GARRETT, ed. *Population, Evolution and Birth Control*. San Francisco: W. H. Freeman and Co. Publishers, 1969.

HAUSER, PHILIP M., ed. *The Population Dilemma*. Englewood Cliffs, N.J.: Prentice-Hall, Inc., 1963.

NG, LARRY K., *The Population Crisis*. Bloomington: Indiana University Press, 1966.

PADDOCK, PAUL and WILLIAM. *Famine, 1975!* Boston: Little, Brown and Company, 1967.

YOUNG, LOUISE B., ed. *Population in Perspective*. New York: Oxford University Press, 1968.

POLLUTION

CURTIS, RICHARD and ELIZABETH HOGAN. *Perils of the Peaceful Atom: The Myth of Safe Nuclear Power Plants*. Garden City, N. Y.: Doubleday & Company, Inc., 1969.

DUBOS, RENÉ. *Man Adapting*. New Haven: Yale University Press, 1967.

EHRLICH, PAUL R. and ANNE H. *Population, Resources, Environment: Issue in Human Ecology*. San Francisco: W. H. Freeman and Co., Publishers, 1970.

GRAHAM, FRANK JR. *Disaster by Default. Politics and Water Pollution.* New York: M. Evans and Company, Inc., 1966.
HERSH, SEYMOUR M. *Chemical and Biological Warfare.* Garden City, N. Y.: Doubleday (Anchor Books), 1969.
LEWIS, HOWARD R. *With Every Breath You Take.* New York: Crown Publishers, Inc., 1965.
MARINE, GENE. *America the Raped.* New York: Simon & Schuster, 1969.
STILL, HENRY. *The Dirty Animal.* New York: Hawthorn Books, Inc., 1967.

GENERAL
COMMONER, BARRY. *Science and Survival.* New York: The Viking Press, 1967.
DE BELL, GARRETT, ed. *The Environmental Handbook.* New York: Ballantine Books, Inc., 1970.
DUBOS, RENÉ. *So Human an Animal.* New York: Charles Scribner's Sons, 1968.
JOHNSON, CECIL E., ed. *Social and Natural Biology.* Princeton, N. J.: D. Van Nostrand Company, Inc., 1968.
MALTHUS, THOMAS R. *An Essay on the Principle of Population as It Affects the Future Improvement of Society, with Remarks on the Speculations of Mr. Godwin, M. Condorcet and Other Writers.* London: Printed for J. Johnson in St. Paul's Church Yard, 1798.
TAYLOR, GORDON R. *The Biological Time Bomb.* New York: World Publishing Co., 1968.
WHYTE, WILLIAM H. *The Last Landscape.* Garden City, N. Y.: Doubleday & Company, Inc., 1968.

Index